Appetite

Also by Karen Throssell
The Old King
Remembering How To Cry
Chain of Hearts
Motherhood Statement
The crime of not knowing your crime – Ric Throssell against ASIO
The Dialectics of Rain
Angles (with Carmel Macdonald Grahame)

Karen Throssell

Appetite
The Politics of Food

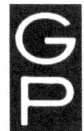

Appetite: The Politics of Food
ISBN 978 1 76109 654 9
Copyright © text Karen Throssell 2023
Cover image: Bry Throssell

First published 2023 by
GINNINDERRA PRESS
PO Box 3461 Port Adelaide 5015
www.ginninderrapress.com.au

Contents

Voracious (1)	7
The Equation	9
Cheaper than therapy and you get zucchini	11
Asparagus	14
Modern Food Foraging	16
Wasn't Time always (our) Precious?	22
When I'm away I go to markets	24
Competition, a Conversation	28
The Omnivore's Dilemma	29
Seed	33
Watching *The Butchers from Brazil*	36
When diet became Diet	38
Porridge	40
Earth Magic	42
The Staff of life	45
Petit Poulet a la Russe – a family culinary history	48
The recipe said, Two Tomatoes	51
Obesogens	53
Artichoke	55
Don't mention the F word…	58
When I'm away I plan gardens	60
Mango	62
Achieving Blisspoint	64
Jack Spratt	65
Jack Spratt's partner	66
Mushrooms	67
Mere Marmalade Maker	69
Nectarine	72
Gluttony – competing forces	74
Removing the Christ…	77

Comfort Food	81
13 things I've learned from Diets – (and one extra)	84
The Peasants – Spuds and Cabbage	86
Spoon Feeding	90
Voracious (2)	93

Voracious (1)

We live in the heart of a beast – Jose Marti

We live in the belly of a beast –
Lives on profits and always hungry

A Midas beast, all he touches
Becomes a Commodity

Even the stuff of life – our food,
We grow what feeds *him*, not what we need

To appease him we must consume and consume
Greed is good: several courses, afters, befores…

I want it all and I want it now
Don't like it, chuck it. The beast loves waste

To fill his fat belly we grow more and more
Pesticides, fungicides and we're eating it all

Give them what they love, and hey, it's addictive!
Why does it even need to be food?

Sugar salt fat, they keep coming back
Fat sugar salt, with plastic toy, petrol voucher

To please him we must accumulate:
Says Moses and the profits*

Swallow the small guy, swallow the farms,
Swallow the forests, the fish

Accumulate! Exterminate! Peach groves in Shepparton
Cheaper from China, buy bulk, sell cheap…

They tumble and roll, tumble and roll
into the coffers of Woolies and Coles

No flavour, no smell, but our Beast has no taste…
Greed and Waste, greed and waste

But they sow the seeds of his destruction.

* Karl Marx wrote in *Das Capital* that the ultimate goal of capitalism is not production but accumulation (Accumulate… Moses and the prophets) is a phrase he uses ironically quoting the scriptures. He also said 'Capitalism sows within itself the seeds of its own destruction.'

The Equation

It's about energy, the in and the out. Too much /too little upsets the balance: Too fat, too thin, obese, starving…

In the *Siege** they nibbled
their daily 125 calories to coincide with
the minimal energy needed to shuffle
to the bakery, to the lake for water
or firewood, lying down after
to conserve what was left…

In the comfortable West
we 've forgotten the equation
we eat for pleasure
and yes it's sublime…
and for us here – one of the easiest
most reliable sources of pleasure
(chocolate more predictable than sex…)

Food as product, constant consumption
chemists, servos, nurseries, bookshops
sausage sizzles outside Bunnings
vending machines in offices, hospitals, stations
snax nibbles afters befores
a drink and nibble before you drink and eat

So much energy making so much money…
the temptress and the torturer –
the telling-us-how-to-look industries:
diet, exercise
fashion, health food

Tweak the equation – denial as power
emaciated girl disguised as fat jumper
marching fast, uphill and down
using the energy from half a cup
of blueberries she had for breakfast
consuming it as soon as it's eaten

What about taste buds?
there to help us distinguish
between bitter/poison, food/horse-shit
or dopamine? There to ensure we eat
to survive so those who can –
eat for pleasure

But we're not children with our little ids
driven entirely by the pleasure principle
we grow up – develop super-ego
self-control, wisdom, balance
some of us learn our equations
or try

* *The Siege* by Helen Dunmore is a fictionalised account of the lives of the people of Leningrad as Hitler attempts to eliminate them by blockading the city and starving them to death.

Cheaper than therapy and you get zucchini

Hands in the earth, humous and worms
all that rotting and renewing…

We remember the cycle – can be with death
acknowledge its contribution to continuing…

Six of us over the years,
all ex-coupled – partners now dead

except Val and hers went off
with his secret Maori lover…

Before she was forced out
Val painted *Bastard* in red, on the wall

of the house where her daughter was born
and which they now had to leave…

*

Between us, we've had:
one die young and sudden in his armchair with his paper

A hero burned to death in bushfire
being brave, 'having to save' his home

A new husband with prostate cancer
(they married after the diagnosis)

Another hero to his union members, a gambler
who killed himself in his car with a hose

An older partner kidnapped by venal kids
who let him die on their watch

An unlamented abuser who was kicked out
and drank himself to death

So much anger amongst the grief
Widows – tearing weeds and heaving mulch

*

We are lucky, as widows go
Still in the 'family home'

with the large garden we'd made together
for that lifetime we'd share…

That garden now in danger of being
a mere reminder of how hard it is:

One person alone, the other the strong one
(physically at least…) left with absence, anguish

*

So do we 'downsize' to a neat unit?
so little maintenance, so easy to clean…

a tub of lavender by the door, then garage
front door, lavender, garage

front door, lavender, garage
door, lavender, garage   Nooooo!

Some do move away, memories left
to languish in old unkempt gardens

But none to a unit! God forbid!
We love our green too much

*

We heal in our new and old gardens
clearing, smoothing, planting, tending

All those symbols – tending our wounds
memories as mulch, nourishing new lives

And we do it together! The power of the collective!
What four women can do in two hours…

Together we can tackle most of the 'boy jobs'
and did we really ever need them?

Some more than others. Maybe need's the wrong word…
And despite vestigial anger and some bad memories

most of us have a special place in our gardens
which we tend alone, on anniversaries…

Asparagus

young shoots of the cultivated lily
like English crocus breaking through winter gloom
you long for them as much as blossom, wattle,
and the feel of warm on sun-starved skin

the most delicious of vegetables
(A, C, B12, potassium, iron)
wickedly phallic unwavering
stalk, and sculpted tips putting carrots
cucumbers, and parsnips to shame

the tips should be lightly furled, perky
rather than limp, and the shoots should be
straight and firm

and so easy – slight steam, dab of butter
twist of pepper, or slice of prosciutto and dob of feta
lends delicate flavour to soufflés, soups
or a spring salad with snow peas broad beans,
watercress and a sprinkle of hazel nuts
or the 'bring-a-plate special' – good old Aussie
asparagus rolls – rolled in white bread with real butter

dad grew it in our canberra garden
up near the compost next to the apricot
with that summer alcohol brown rot smell…
called it the magic pudding plant
cut and come again all spring
until it announces its retirement
by transforming into a feathery hedge

as a kid I was only interested in the autumn
red berries peeping through the soft green
and I don't think I ever ate it
I only knew it as tinned – dark, soggy and bitter

maybe mum didn't know how –
preferred things frozen or in cans
much more modern for the fifties housewife
maybe we tried it and turned up our noses
had beans instead while mum and dad
had the grown-up feast

now, every spring I make up for lost time…

Modern Food Foraging

Hunting for bargains and gathering packaging

Interviewer

Eating is a lot like breathing. Absolutely vital to life, but taken for granted.

We know that what we put into our bodies keeps us alive. We seem to understand less that the quality of what we put in, equally affects the quality of our life – and by quality of life we don't mean overseas trips and outdoor kitchens – we mean optimum health.

Why then are we content to put stuff into our bodies that is further and further removed from real food? Stuff that is manufactured and sold by companies that are exclusively profit driven.

Yes, exclusively. They don't give a toss about the nutritional value of what makes money. In fact they don't care if it's actually harmful to our health as a lot of it is. So they think: easy (chemicals, additives) attractive (artificial colours, packaging advertising) and addictive (sugar salt fat, and chemicals) accessible (put it all in the one place with all the most addictive and unnecessary items at eye and hand level – chocolates biscuits snacks) with parking close by, and as cheap as they can, while maintaining maximum profit.

So why do we eat 'food' that not only doesn't do us any good, it positively does us bad?

You know the answer – sugar salt fat, convenience, time and cost.

But I shouldn't be answering the questions. I set out to find what others think.

Interviews

Denise
It's my Scottish blood. Cost is the factor. Top quality for bottom dollar. I do believe in the value of organic produce. I don't doubt that we're better off having chemically free food. But there's absolutely no way I'm going to pay double for it.

Karly
We had an organic food shop here for a while and everybody loved the idea. There were three of us in the room when we found out that it had gone broke and was closing down. 'That's terrible' we all said. But we all also said that we hardly ever shopped there – none of us could afford to buy the produce.
$11 for a cauliflower! I just couldn't do it!

Interviewer

But is it really too expensive?

'A perception of organic food as an elite privilege is a considerable obstacle to the farmer growing food for middle-income customers whose highest food-shopping priority is the lowest price. Growing food without polluting the field or the produce will always cost more than the conventional mode that externalises costs to the tax payer and the future.

It is interesting that penny-pinching is an accepted defence for toxic food habits, when frugality so rarely rules other consumer domains. At any income level we can be relied upon for categorically unnecessary purchases: portable earplug music instead of the radio (and the latest one every year when the other one is still working perfectly); extra fast internet for leisure use; heavy vehicles to transport light loads; name brand clothing new every season.'

(*Animal, Vegetable, Miracle*, Barbara Kingsolver, Faber & Faber 2007)

Denise
I only ever buy dairy, cans, biscuits, deli at the supermarket. I've found a good butcher, and there's a good fish shop in Ringwood.

Deborah
We don't like the quality of the meat and fish from the supermarket. My husband does the meat shopping – he has a particular butcher that he likes.

Pam
I do the supermarket. Rob does the butcher. He gets on so well with him that when we went overseas, Rob sent him a T-shirt.

Denise
Dad became so friendly with our butcher that he used to make soup for them and take it over for their lunch. When he died, they closed the shop and attended the funeral.

Pam
And of course supermarkets make it so much easier. You don't have to go to separate shops – butchers, bakers, greengrocers. It's all there in the one big shop, all on the same docket. You only have to use your card once. What could be easier? And you've got underground parking, trolley to the car. And these days with time being so precious, you've got to do it.

Interviewer

But what about taste? Surely this is as important if not more so than convenience and cost. Most people who try it, say organic food grown close to home taste heaps better (even if it often looks less perfectly formed and shiny.

Deborah
I stopped buying vegies from the supermarket three years ago. I got sick of bringing celery home that was limp by the time I got there. And it had no taste. We grow a lot of our own now. It makes such a difference. I remember my first cauliflower – stunted little thing it was. But it tasted delicious. It was like rediscovering its flavour.

Aaron
I used to be the local butcher. I was sure it would work here. Nice little community with a bit of money around, so they would appreciate quality. When I heard they'd fought against the supermarket, and fought again when it tried to take over some of the small shops, I was sure it was right. They'd welcome me with open arms. They'd love my perfect little noisettes, cutlets 'frenched' like the supermarket have never heard of, beautiful fresh meat,

butchered by a pro, not like those hacked plastic slabs where you'd hardly know what animal it was from. I can't believe that's what people think meat is. So god, I don't know. Here I am, broke – after a year and a half. My wife pregnant again, probably have to sell the house to pay off my debts. Supermarket wins again – the triumph of big business!

Pam
But these days with time being so precious, you've got to do it.

Aaron
All those hard years as a fucking apprentice, nearly lost two fingers, wallowing in blood and guts half the day. But I was bloody good, the meat was bloody good, as good as they'd ever get and the bloody cretins couldn't see. They just couldn't see…

We know about the economies of scale
vegies at supermarkets always on sale
They buy huge quantities all year round.
Small farmers miseries just compound

Wasn't Time always (our) Precious?

Precious / of great value because rare expensive important minutes hours days glint alluringly / diamond seconds minutes / silver weeks months / golden years decades / but unlike jewels once they're gone / they're gone forever

Time is money / is our invention /our creation / 'Greenwich Mean Time' / separate units seconds minutes hours days week months years seasons / meaningful to the market / society slots in

So there's the 24-hour day / oh and of course / *8 hours work rest and play* / but does it count if unpaid / housework and childcare / do we count the commute / voluntary work / unpaid overtime / so that neatly divided day not so neat after all

Is when the market / controls most of our day / when time is most precious? working families / clock on / bell rings / don't miss the bus pick up the kids / clean house cook dinner wash up iron clothes sleep / what's sleep? / and play? those precious jewels winking away / not enough *time* / other things sacrificed / yes of course / all those housekeeping chores/ / what is essential anyway?

Scarce time / also more visible / first smile first tooth first step / no longer newborn baby toddler child prepubescent adolescent / watching / time strokes /clock ticks / tock tick time so vital / must not be wasted

Wasting time / is it wasted when we spend it / is one negative
the other positive / and each as subjective/ as humans are
complex / *Examined life* / *Carpe Diem* / *live each day as if it's
your last* / weighing up

For some / growing and cooking / delicious nutritious
defying the non-food / produce not products / nurturing the
earth / nourishing the children / spending not wasting
fruitfully pleasurably / a 'lifestyle' even

For others / so many time-saving options / takeaway
restaurants Uber Eats! / cheap packaged frozen meals / tins
packets / all that free time / to do other / more useful
important relaxing and fun things

When we seem / to have a lot more / *on our hands* / even
more precious / as in running out / when the big R hits
gleefully dolefully / no longer regulated / by capital's clock
even worse / our own clock's ticking / tock tick / all those
lovely time-strokes / of our growing children / suddenly no
longer welcomed / time measured / by our increasingly
obvious / mortality / then it becomes / vital / to use every
minute / of what we have left / wisely:

Time to / nourish teach learn / fulfil goals / support values
give us pleasure give others pleasure / truly and finally
treasuring our Precious…

When I'm away I go to markets

Now when I'm a guest I don't usually ferret
through friend's fridges
but hungry and left to my own devices
or offering to cook because it's 7 p.m.
and there's no sign of action…

This fridge is like a student's or bachelor's
without the beer: one carrot, half an onion
shredded brown-tipped iceberg lettuce
and the tiniest broccoli floret
which I thought was a sprig of parsley –
Each item in its own snap-lock bag…

Julie hates to cook, and isn't interested
in anything but getting her nourishment
the easiest way. Obsessed with low calories
the cupboard is full of no-cook options:
four bean mixes, tinned tuna, soups
and non-food in boxes and packets:

Tandaco One-pan dinner (just add meat)
Amy's split pea soup – organic, low fat and gluten free
Kraft Mac and Cheese 'piles and piles of smiles'
(My daughter had a version when she was young
called 'Easi-Mac' which looked like glue
and smelled like vomit)

Like walking into a room
where no one speaks your language
and they all turn their backs…
I flee to a local market to hear some English
Ah! It was like being surrounded by friendly
voices – exuberant yet soothing, joyous yet reflective
and some of it was Italian…

A cornucopia of colour!
Red green orange yellow purple puce
tumbling in voluptuous mounds begging to be
stroked, squeezed, sniffed. Ripe apricots
mangoes, peaches cupped in ecstasy,
breathed in – eyes closed…

Each seem to compete – *look at me, look at me*
the glossiest fat purple aubergines
palely orange polished persimmons
the pink blush on new season pears
and tomatoes, in multi-shades
of red orange yellow blue (Russian)
Glowing sun-jewels

Then there was the meat section:
vac-wrapped slabs of pale fat-white pink
or dried-blood brown… The colour of death
You would have to become a vego
if only on aesthetic grounds

I turned to the colour and filled my basket
When all stacked in the fridge
or in bowls on benches
it felt like home…

Pommes d'Amour

Why are they the missiles thrown
at the unpopular by the hostile?
Because they are meant to be soft and squashy
Small red juice bombs that can splat, squish, plop
Make a big mess down the front of white shirts

They're nightshade, of course there's wicked potential
(with the evil aubergine, creepy capsicum
and that petulant potato)
Or fun! – A *pomme d'amour* – love apple
succulent crimson flesh splits and spills
Really a fruit – plump and sweet
Gran served them with sugar for dessert
said it was strange to add pepper and salt
But some tomatoes need no sugar
Summer tomatoes, the fruit of love

Winter tomatoes, Clayton's tomatoes –
These *pommes-de-mort*
could never muster the passion
to invite flinging – for a cause
It would be like throwing rocks

You could kill someone

Competition, a Conversation

Money, media, lawyers and pollies, all stacked against us.
But it's just a big shop! It needs us more than we need…
So bloody big it needs to shout it, Now it's BIG (friendly) W
so BIG you feel helpless, so huge you get lost…

So here it is – *Accumulation* –
Sucking them up or sending them broke:
grocers and butchers, bakers and milk bars,
florists and delis fatten it up…

But there's still competition! We're no Evil Empire:
– only one soap brand, grey queues for sameness
We have 'free markets' and 63 brands
And yes competition… There's always Big C

And with one of them looming, the small shops, the locals
are forced to shut down, sucking the soul
from lost country towns. They straddle
whole blocks – just them and the pub –

Hang on a minute, they own the pubs too
'Family fun' means poker machines –
machines based on greed, and for cheating the desperate.
Money for nothing and your drinks for free

But old Karl was right about seeds of destruction.
Who cares about size, with the strength of those seeds?

*The Omnivore's Dilemma**

We're top of the food chain
Of course it's our right.
Our bodies designed for it
Part of our culture…

> *Succulent pieces of beef*
> *slowly braised with bacon,*
> *mushrooms, a good shiraz,*
> *and a splosh of cream*

Completely natural
Look at our canines
Precisely there for the tearing of flesh
And we need the protein…

> But I won't eat anything:
> that has a face
> that is really cute
> that I've given a name

>> *Roast sliced Jerusalem artichokes*
>> *with thyme and lemon. Fry cherry*
>> *tomatoes till they collapse. Serve*
>> *with basil oil and fried halloumi*

> I will eat it, if it's had a happy life
> eating organic food in fresh air
> its natural death, painless
> and peaceful

I don't eat cows or old sheep
when I pass them grazing
contented, in the field –
You're safe from me

> *Caramelise red onions and garlic*
> *Stir in cinnamon, cumin, paprika*
> *coriander. Stir into cooked lentils*
> *and top with spring onions*

I say, averting my eyes from
lambs and piglets explaining
I won't eat them if I can recognise
flesh that has frolicked

> *A large bunch of fresh basil*
> *Several cloves of garlic, pine nuts*
> *or walnuts salt and pepper. Blitz*
> *with olive oil. Add grated parmesan*

Only if they are mixed with
fennel, salt, sodium nitrate or genuinely
smoked and turned into 'charcuterie'
will I eat them

And I do detest the way they are treated –
battery chickens, feedlot cows
force-fed geese, and sheep killed live
But what can we do?

> *Tender pink spring lamb*
> *flavoured with garlic,*
> *rosemary, lemon,*
> *and eucalypt smoke*

Without mass production
who'd feed the world?
They need the protein
We help the masses

> *Crispy roast chicken running*
> *with golden juices, flavoured*
> *with lemon, bacon, tarragon*

Of course it's our right
Our bodies designed for it
It's part of our culture
We're top of the food chain

> *Eat food*
> *Not too much*
> *Mainly from plants**

---

* Michael Pollan – *The Omnivore's Dilemma*

Farms that survive are really vast
The family farm a thing of the past
agribusinesses is now the go
mono-crops is what they grow:

Seed

I remember warm dark days
before-days, when comfort-coiled
I waited for signs – drips of damp
tempting my tightness. Slowly I unfold
stretch. Now I know there is an Up
to aim for. I straighten, thrust…
Suddenly this burst of bright!
Mother releases me

Now this was never part of the deal…
Just going about my business
with sun and rain – my perfect green slow-grow.
So what's this on the wind?
The devil's mad brew?
Too fast, too tall, all show
roots can't support – goodness all gone
Mother won't be pleased

And here is her vengeance
Think you can bend me to your will?
Screw you, and your poisonous greed
She groans, roars and cracks
wide open, gaping wound to be plugged
by you and all your detritus
But who will survive her wrath? Why me!
She is mother – I am reborn

Perfect Persimmon

Diospyros – Divine fruit

Orange oozy sumptuousness
skin-sliding off like a skun rabbit
(but the cheery orange stops you
balking at the comparison)
appeals to your inner messy kid, who wallows
in sloppy squelchy chin-dripping food
which no one can eat and keep themselves clean

Defies all the rules of 'fresh off the tree'
Actually has to sit on the sill till its old
and squashy enough to be sweet
Too early and it's puckering sour –
So – a fruit which is perfect
when it's wrinkled and ancient
Gives you a new perspective on aging

A divinely beautiful fruit, Bright shiny
apricot tones – glowing as it ripens on the ledge
perfect sunset globes gracing the tree's naked arms.
Just for the artists, it ripens after leaf fall
Much painted, printed and etched, in its native
Japan – you'd plant it for that art in your garden

Male and female flowers grow on separate trees
But sometimes there's a special tree:
both male and female, pink and creamy white
making a 'perfect' hermaphrodite
So it doesn't need its 'other half'
Gives you a new perspective on we spinsters…

In Ozark folklore it can predict
the severity of the coming winter
In Korea the dried persimmon has
a reputation for scaring away tigers
In our folklore it could be a symbol
of exquisite and succulent
mature spinsterhood

Watching *The Butchers from Brazil**

Thinking Brazil – corrupt colonels
steaming *favelas,* burning rainforests
gangsters with hatchets

The Batista brothers – different butchers
Exploiting the real ones
Murder minus machetes

Corrupt as any colonels, buying and bribing
across the world. Baby-faced billionaires
No striped aprons for them…

The butcher brothers, adept at carving
meat empires. Chopping into
the small guys callously culling family

butchers   local abattoirs
And yes! Hacking and slashing
the beleaguered

rainforests, clearing the way for cattle to graze,
fatted for slaughter. All the better for
the mass meat market

They've long tight tentacles – they're even in OZ…
squeezing Aldis, Woolies, Coles, as far as
The Apple Isle – 'Tassie salmon' lies at their feet

Their workers ground up and spat out
wages trimmed, *get rid of that fat*
safety, security   into the bin
The Batista boys – Accumulate   Accumulate!
Flesh on the floor and money
in the bloody pocket

* *The Butchers from Brazil, Four Corners,* May 2022

When diet became Diet
when we turned from produce to Product

Once our diet was in our gardens
We ate what we produced
Food was for nourishment, it kept us alive
Protein, fat, carbohydrate, fibre
All do important things
Balance, was the answer

Now we have Shoulds and Should nots
'Experts' and 'Science' – A triangle that inverts
The good becomes bad and back again
Every year a new Diet,
Every month a new Fad:

Robert Atkins (all protein) Fit for Life (don't mix carbs and protein) Low GI (eat every 2 hours) Gluten Free (no bread or pasta), Mediterranean (eat like a Greek) Israeli (eat grapefruit – they look like bombs, and you can steal all the water) Paleo (eat like a cave dweller – protein and fat but no carbs, what about when here are no mammoths?) 5/2 Fasting (hardly eat at all for 2 out of 5 days, pig out on the others.) NOOM ('but it's)not a diet' – divide food into colours and have daily counselling 'FOD Map (Eat bugger all but Bone Broth) KETO (this era's Atkins with a few tweaks, because Robert Atkins died of a heart attack.)

Food now not just part of life – but a huge source of
Angst, consternation, contradiction…
Don't eat fat/ meat/sugar/carbs/ protein/grains/ and pulses
Eat just protein; eat just carbs; all grains and pulse
Fat's OK, eat more but only if it's good fat…only if it's 'natural',
But vegetables stay safe don't they?
No! Some are high in GI
Some are Carbs! Some don't fit on FODMap
Fruit? No! All that fructose…

The poor old spud is regularly bad – high in gluten and peptins
Sugar stays consistent – empty calories, super-addictive
But it shows us what happened:
When we ate what we grew
Sugar – a treat, in a cake for a birthday
Or in wine for a feast

Then the merchants slink in
They know it's addictive
It's in all their products –
Even the savoury ones…
Making us buy/eat more and more

The real Diet is the Product Diet
Products not produce make Profits!
diet Diet Die!

Porridge

Frost-filled mist-shrouded mornings
and you hate leaving
your downy haven
toasty feet feel freeze of slate floor
grope for woolly Uggs – Aaargh…
But it's the soaking oats
gets you out of your cocoon

Add milk, raisins
Turn stove and heater on low
Scuttle back to bed for a snug half hour
Then when you've heard the news
and planned your day

your oats will be thick and creamy
Add honey, chopped autumn-sweet apple
and sigh. Tummy full and warm
you can now admire the misty hills
the beauty of frost sparkling spiderwebs
and start your day

*

Discovered by Scots and Swiss
where oats, more than wheat or maize
survived freezing boglands, frozen Alps…
They say Scots soldiers served
it with a slosh of whisky for extra warmth

In Switzerland, a bag of oats
was tied around the cow's neck
fed both herder and herd
The Swiss later developed
a summer version – muesli!

From the solid sustenance
of the working class, to the current day
when served with with goji berries, chia
and oat milk, it is the food of choice for
healthy hipsters and pampered poets

Earth Magic

In a world in which the life of the soil is under assault, building soil fertility can be a profound act of worship

I love my compost. This wonderful pile
of slimy mould ridden not-waste
seething with flies and grubs

shape-shifting into lumpy brown, finally
running through your fingers chocolate rich
and full of goodness

like the Magic Pudding:
steak and kidney, with a pot for a hat
and a bad temper…

once sliced, grows itself again
a perennial pudding!
and even it can't turn back into a cow…

the cycle of fertility and decay…
means compost does!
rotting layers, slowly

disintegrate construct renew
less and less you see
old dead food, eggshells, orange peel

mouldy clots of sludge disappear
turn grassier then browner
swarming with the myriad creatures

it is feeding, who are feeding it
ants and worms and beetles
and the thin threads, long arms of *mycorrhizal fungi**

compost is
>Poetry – ordinary becomes extraordinary
>Chemistry – nitrogen/carbon combining, reacting. creating
>Religion – rotting plants/*earth*; sun/*fire;* rain/*water*; wind/*air*,
>Alchemy – the ancient art of transformation

* *mycorrhizal* fungi that unpack the nutrients in rocks and decomposing soil

Pesticides sprayed from light planes
Monsanto spewed for maximum gain
Killing off the insect world
Eco disaster they've unfurled

The Staff of life

Back then it was every meal
A 'heel 'with a stew
or a chunk of cheese
Dense brown crusty
you had to rip it with your teeth
Stale the next day
If it lasted that long

The secret was your yeast
your wild yeast, 'caught'
like wayward thoughts, carried
on a cloud. Flour and water in a jar
taken somewhere special –
a smooth stone by a quiet river
Leave overnight with a loose lid

Wild yeast spins in the wind
there for the catching in moonlight
A micro-organism that feeds on
carbohydrate, releases carbon dioxide
when you open your jar – it's bubbling
it's yours, there to share as it
beautifully doubles – the more it makes
the more you give…

Give! Voracious won't be pleased

It turned white when 'refined'
like those who could afford it…
Remember *Heidi* who stole*
white rolls from rich folks
Which she thought would cure
her sick cousin? Of course it was
the fresh mountain air that did it!

And now the reversal:
Only the rich in time can bake their own
Only the rich in money can afford
the 'hand made artisan loaf'
The ubiquitous white sliced wettex
is for the masses
They've removed the bran and fibre – why?

Ask Voracious!

He wants Modern bread,
grown with dwarf wheat –
Fast growing, high yielding…
Plus fertiliser – higher and faster

Modern bread, made with synthetic yeast
Fast rising, high rising
Plus additives – even higher even faster

And because 'white is good'
and whiter is better
you add bleach and bromide

Cheap production   high turnover   higher sales
Fast Profits   Faster profits   Even faster profits…
'
    All together now!   (to the tune of 'This Land is Your Land')†
        They don't eat food here
        They just eat plastic
        They make their bread from
        compressed elastic
        They eat what is good for GNP*

---

*Heidi – children's book by Johanna Spyri written in 1881, ranked with the Bible and Shakespeare as one of the world's most widely read books.
† from 'This Land is Your Land', it's sure not my land – by KT 1973 with apologies to Pete Seeger

Petit Poulet a la Russe – a family culinary history

Mama hated cooking –
was never taught, her mother didn't care
Mama was an artist, lived in Paris once
ate her meals in smoky cafés
with *beaucoup du vin rouge*[1]

In another life we ate her wifely fare:
chops carrots peas, sausages and mash
Friday fish, and frozen chips
But Father cooked on Sundays: Pasta! Rice!
'Curry' with coconut, bananas

Fussy younger siblings soon began to whinge:
They said the food was strange
Dad sulked, took away his whisk and bowl
Mama was annoyed. She didn't get to go on strike
because customers complained

Now our grandma was a cook
She'd been to Russia, brought back
Petit Poulet a la Russe: chicken, bacon[2]
almonds, asparagus. No cabbage, dumplings?
More Français than Russe…

She showed how much she loved us
with little gifts of food – beside our breakfast
plates when we came to stay:
jams from her garden – fig for Dad, apricot for me
and for Mum, her golden Cape gooseberry

Her special porridge:
Apples, honey, dates, wheatgerm.
(Remember wheatgerm?)
Health food before her time
she and Gaylord Hauser.[3]

Petit Poulet du Mama had[4]
bacon rolls with toothpicks
almonds from a packet, asparagus from a tin
the whole thing swamped in white sauce
A glug of sherry – *her je ne sais quoi.*[5]

Foods of the World arrived – the first one – *France*
Time-Life changed our lives. Dad sneered. Yanks?
teaching us to cook! But I was hooked:
picnics with paté, baguettes, brie
meals of soufflés, crepes, quiche…

Mama was delighted, though perplexed
Could not understand the fuss
My *Petit Poulet:* fresh asparagus, prosciutto
chicken breasts – marinated, chargrilled
A vodka toast: *Salut La Russe!*

The dish moves on once more, to France
My daughter cooks it her way when I stay –
asparagus and almonds from her garden…
She enfolds it all in pastry, adds camembert and cream,
She's a vego now, it's become *sans poulet!*[6]

1 *beaucoup du vin rouge* –lots of red wine
2 G. Hauser – health food guru, popular in the 1950, promoted yoghurt, molasses, and wheatgerm…
3 *petit poulet a la Russe* – little chicken in the Russian style
4 *du Mama* – Mama's version
5 *je ne sais quoi* – a mysterious special touch
6 *sans poulet* – without chicken

The recipe said, *Two Tomatoes*

And I thought Red…
passionate, cloak swirling red
tomato-red for god's sake
soft, succulent
oozing with summer
still fragrant, warm
cupped in your hand

Picked straight off the vine
dripping onto your bare feet then
mixed with sweet-perfumed basil
fruity green olive oil
a touch of garlic
a shave of cheese –
Aaah tomatoes…

But it is August!
grey, soggy freezing August
the time of ghost tomatoes
pretend tomatoes
hard, pale dry tomatoes
picked green, screaming
Not yet, not yet…

Grown in hot houses
with cold wet windows
never knowing the feel of
sun warming their flesh
gently giving their skin
a deeper and deeper glow.

I've heard they can make them square
to fit better on square bread.
That's why they like them juiceless
so they don't make the bread soggy
Better for all the thousands
of miles they have to travel

So, I dumped the recipe
bought some leeks
Kinglake fresh, pulled yesterday
earth just shaken off
sweet and butter succulent
Loving that cold earth
warm, hearty – winter

Obesogens

Ultra-processed foods are the major contributor to childhood obesity and child diabetes, as well as the alarming rate of obesity in the general population of most Western countries

A large oval table with water and mints
Power Point presentations by serious men
Grey suited, tied down, important business
But what are these bowls placed down the middle?
Are they really piles of Krispy Kremes?

It's not an excessive morning tea
for the unreconstructed, nor leftovers
from the tubby kids' party
It is a vital work of *product improvement*
A search for *hyper-palatability*

Each man reaches out, takes
a slow thoughtful bite
giving those earnest wine tasters
a run for their money
One says, Not sweet enough *add more sugar*

Another says, Not crispy enough *add more fat*
Not moist in the centre – *must fix that mouth feel*
Not moreish enough *MSG, PHA, BHT*
A bit more of this, a touch more of that…

Finally they all nod—
Just Right!
We've achieved Blisspoint!

A meeting of drug peddlers
working on the perfect equation
for maximum addiction
Starting with those controlled by their ids,
who haven't yet learned about food as guilt

In a world where we expect *to have it all
and have it now,* we start with the kids
Sugar salt fat they keep coming back
playing with their little brains
Why eat porridge when you have pop tarts?

What do they call chemicals
that create maximum deliciousness
maximum moreishness?
Obesogens

Artichoke

Sunchoke, Earth Apple, Sunflower

The first time is at *Petty Sessions*
Dinner with Dad at a posh restaurant
You must try the special – Artichoke soup!
I know you'll love it. I certainly do…

Where has this wonder been all my life?
Rare as truffles, caviar, crayfish?
No! They're so easy to grow
they're not worth a thing

And they're a bit anti-social,
they're called farty-chokes!
Only a problem in 'polite society'
Dad says with a grin…

Such yummy food shunned
for this small felony?
Like cream and sugar despite the taste?
or caffeine and grog despite their therapy?

Yes, and yes, the slim, healthy scream
But that's so long-term. I relish the now
The poor artichoke can bloat you a bit
might make you 'windy – just stay out of lifts

But highly nutritious –
potassium, iron, fibre of course…
diabetes' folk medicine
and completely delicious:

Nutty and sweet (big dose of fructose)
Hints of sesame, truffle
cool crunch of chestnut
sweet and earthy at the same time

like fat knobs of ginger or small warty spuds
dirt crammed in their creases
hopeless to peel –
weird shapes confuse peelers

It becomes all too hard
We want it uniform, packaged
pre-washed and cut
chemically treated to deal with the gut

But you then miss the joy
of scrabbling in soil, feeling them down there
snuggling in clusters, blinking at sunlight
The deeper you go, the bigger they are

And for a new crop next autumn
you just leave a few…
Not too many, they'll quickly take over
Exuberant, generous in every way

Then you scrub and you trim
make shapes you can peel
cook with butter and garlic or bake with tomatoes
top with thyme and halloumi or

a big pot of soup with bacon and celery
à la Petty Sessions
They gave me the recipe –
treasured for years

I eat them all autumn
by myself

Don't mention the F word…

It was her aged face I noticed
Peculiarly lined for one so young
Eighteen or eighty…
Wrinkles carved across her forehead
Hard lines etched from nose to chin –

Worse when she smiled
Skin stretched so tight it could crack
Like the wizened masks of
Tiny babies with old men's faces
Africa, India…starvation masks

Her body explains it –
Impossibly frail, arms so thin
You wonder how she lifts her tray
Her grasshopper legs encased in
Thick black tights in the summer heat

What is she thinking as she serves us lunch?
Aromas of bacon, garlic, warm bread, coffee?
Hammering on that hollow stomach which in a day
Has only had three spoons of no-fat yoghurt.
Oblivious to aroma — she abhors the F word.

Its not Africa and famine
But affluent Australia,
and self-inflicted
Look at me, I am beautiful
And I'm so in control…

Fresh, family run, flavoursome friendly
Or
Foolish futile fairies (away with the…)

When I'm away I plan gardens

I dream of green profusion
tight bright clumps, spidery tendrils
big floppy leaves, feathery fronds sprawling
Tucked in are sweet parsnips, and small crunchy carrots

But here are these pale fridge replicas.
Sad little soldiers laid out on black slabs
cling-wrap straight-jacket pulled tight to hide
colourless sag, and what are these huge pinkish things?

Grapefruit large – for fitting
one slice per sandwich
square dry tomatoes
for mess-free convenience
>*seeds compost sun rain*
>*green thrust sun shoots*
>*strong plant strong roots*
>*ripe now pick EAT*
>*return to compost*
>*cycle complete*

Think of home and sunny ledges
covered in the last stunted and bird pecked
tomatoes which even though not quite
fresh off the vine still taste of summer

So I draw plans for autumn – neat rows that never behave
dream of earth alchemy – that fruity brew:
cow shit, blood and bone, potash, eye of newt
soon trickling soft and brown through my fingers

Dream of sweet baby carrots pulled from their beds
dusting off dirt and crunching them raw –
steaming a parsnip with a ginger touch
orange peel, butter, black pepper, chives…

> *seeds compost sun rain*
> *green thrust sun shoots*
> *strong plant strong roots*
> *ripe now pick EAT*
> *return to compost*
> *cycle complete*

Whenever I'm home I plant gardens

Mango

They used to be a luxury
our Christmas morning treat
After the presents were opened
we'd line up at the sink or outside
to wallow in the sweetly sloppy mess

Dad was always scathing
about the 'neat' way of eating them
the cross cuts that pushed out cute squares
to pop into your mouth without a drip
He said it was too prissy
like the European way of eating fruit

on a plate with a knife. He called it 'taming'
Taming an apple was bad enough
but taming a mango was sacrilege!
So sensuous, succulent
the golden gorgeous flesh meant for
sucking and slurping
strips getting caught in your teeth
juice running down your chin
between your sticky fingers

One boyfriend at Christmas was
astonished at our mango reverence
He was from Queensland where he said
they were cattle food
They would drop plop off the tree
the cows would eat them
shit out the pips

He had never tried one…

After a solemn tasting,
he said *they were OK
but he preferred a nice crisp apple*
He didn't last long…

Achieving Blisspoint

Our brains are hard-wired to want 'rewarding' When we eat junk foods the reward circuits are activated and release dopamine. The brain gets overwhelmed by these foods and releases more dopamine actually negatively altering how our brains function.

Why do we eat what we know is unhealthy?
Processed food devoid of all good
It alters our brain, so we want more and more
Bypasses our natural feelings of hunger

Processed food doing positive harm
When did our produce become packaged product?
Eating makes money – *don't wait for hunger!*
Chemical agents affect our absorption

When did our produce become packaged product?
Companies work on creating addiction
Chemical agents affect our metabolism
Our brains are hard wired to respond to rewarding

Companies work on creating addiction
Ultra-processed is ultra-addictive
Our brains are hard-wired to respond to rewarding
Food is also adjusted for 'mouth feel'

Ultra-processed is ultra-addictive
It alters our brain, so we want more and more
The perfect equation of salt sugar fat
Why do we eat what we know is unhealthy?

Jack Spratt

Reasons not to eat

beauty
of bones
sparce
scaffolding
clean
uncluttered
I did this!
It is a war
fighting need
I am in control
not my mother
nor the doctor
nor my appetite
or the pushers
with their spells
and chemicals
others need it
to survive
I can survive
without
because
I am
in
control
and
almost
gone

Jack Spratt's partner

Reasons for eating

Bliss
Ecstasy, Pleasure
Hyperpalatabillity, Sugarsaltfat
Make today special! Live for now!
Habit, Security, Comfort
Time for a Kit Kat! Snak Attak!
Consolation, Celebration, *Obesogens, Sugarsaltfat*
Beat the blues! Feed your good! Fuel for Fun!
Self-esteem Peer pressure Depression, Anomie
Achieving Blisspoint, Obesogens MSG
Make mornings Epic! Because you deserve it!
I stretch, crunch have to work hard to be this thin!
Addiction, Obsession, Megarexia
Hyperpalatabillity, Sugarsaltfat
Achieving Blisspoint, Obesogens MSG
Dunkin Donuts, Real Food For
Your Busy Life!
McDonalds, Nutella, Nestle, Coca-Cola
Pass the Heinz! We Love Our Vegemite!
Finger Lickin'good!
Banish Hunger!
Hunger?

Mushrooms

Cento/Conversation with Sylvia Plath

Overnight, very
Whitely, discreetly,
Very quietly

Our toes, our noses
Take hold on the loam
Acquire the air

Shelter with fairies
Who guide us
Navigate magic

Circles whose centres
Grant wishes
Soft fists clench in victory

Or determination
Nudgers and shovers
In spite of ourselves

Apparently *bland-mannered*
We mushrooms morph
With culinary alchemy*

Become meat
For the meat-less
Innocuous white becomes

Dense black with juicy pleats
Pushing pink flesh
Off plates

Your spider-tendrilled sisters†
Deeply subterranean
Web-spread protectors

Together we shall soon
Inherit the earth
Our foot's in the door

* butter, garlic bacon black pepper
† *mycorrihizal* fungi unpack nutrients in decomposing soil

Mere Marmalade Maker

Once a year we'd cross the boiling Nullarbor
to the green oasis of my Gran's house
nestling in the Perth hills

Always waiting at the gate
hopping and twittering with glee
she showered us with love tokens –
                                    Equal amounts of sugar and fruit
A vase of wildflowers beside the bed
a jar of our own special jam
favourites from her garden

Fig for Dad, Cape gooseberry for Mum
chunky syrupy strawberry for me
That first breakfast so special –

outside in her cobbled courtyard
the pergola roof dripping with currants
our own personally labelled jam beside our plates

                                              Add peel for pectin
From the generation where you ate
from your garden, and preserved the excess
when Persephone had retreated to the darkness

and whilst special for us,
it was something one did
Writing was her real love, and she never stopped

                                              Bring to a rolling boil

Dad stopped suddenly. *I've got no more words…*
I'm all written out
The timing was terrible

                                          Spoon onto a cold saucer

A life cramming writing into non-work corners
Such is the fate of our heart's work
in the face of the need to earn…

And now the Big R and those yawning years…
Suddenly you stop being taken seriously
People used to listen. I had some gravitas
                                         Ready when wrinkled if pushed

And such hard carved authority…
No longer senior bureaucrat – merely a SOB
Dad's new acronym – Silly Old Bloke…

                                            Three-fruit Marmalade
So much more than his work persona
Writer, playwright, actor, director…
But when no longer bureaucrat/breadwinner

he dropped all his bundles
became a marmalade maker
Pouring his creative soul into the alchemy of cooking?
                                            Five-fruit Marmalade
No – born in the wrong era
domestic work was not creative!
Just part of his SOB image – Mere Marmalade Maker…

                              Seven-fruit Marmalade
But he delighted in the diversity of citrus   Orange
His glowing gold jars too, became love   Lemon
tokens for visiting adult children   Lime
                                                      Mandarin
We took them to our distant homes when he died   Cumquat
preserving those sweet sour memories…   Grapefruit
I kept the last jar for years   Tangelo

Finally opened with great ceremony
We couldn't eat it
Love's bitter fruit

Nectarine

Special because they insist on their season
though you can get them too early –
hard, small, and (warned by the price tag) tasteless
or strangely sharp, when you're expecting sweet

But never all year – like all those others
who of course have their seasons
but are there all the time
(Ah, the convenience: Whatever you want – Now!)

Fresh off the tree they're a different species
even the ubiquitous apple-a-day
only drippily sweet and deliciously crisp
when the air and the leaves are crisping too

So that first nectarine is extra special
the golden ecstasy of oozy summers
sweet honeyed flesh says:
sleepy afternoons on veranda hammocks

breakfasts on balconies – with fresh milk on muesli
barbecues on beaches – grilled with tabouli
and if there's so many you can bear to cook them
sliced on a flan, with pastry and cream…

I have two nectarine trees
they belong to the parrots
who attack them too early
leave them strewn, mutilated

Desperate for just a taste
I pick a barely soft few
to ripen on ledges
When ripe, they taste a bit like

the bought ones – picked out of season

Gluttony – competing forces

Characterised by a limitless appetite for food and drink, overindulgence to the point where one is no longer eating to live but living to eat…

The Michelin people waddling along
in 'All you can Eat' cafés
Plates piled so high they wobble
like the waddlers

Spoilt fat brat cramming face full of crap
shoving in more and more till puffed cheeks
look like cup cakes

Vast rolling Americans in *The Triplets of Belleville*
Fat man, woman, child
ice cream in one hand hot dog in the other

La Grande Bouffe
eating to die
to stave off anomie

Eating too much is bad for us – health industry
diet Industry bleat. Others bleat – fat shaming!
It's common sense: the Equation –
Eat as much as you need for the energy you expend

But excess is the least of our worries
Gluttony is one of the seven deadlies
The sin of *sensual gratification*

St Gregory the Great
There are many ways to succumb to the sin of gluttony

St Thomas Aquinas
Nimus   excess consumption
Studiose   excessive quality, too dainty or elaborately prepared
Laute   too luxurious, exotic or costly
Praepropere   too hastily consumed, too soon or at the wrong times
Ardente   eating too eagerly

But the Beast says the opposite!
We must
WANT IT ALL AND HAVE IT NOW!

NIMUS

        Cafés offering *All you Can Eat*
        befores afters appetisers entrees
        morning tea afternoon tea drinks
        and nibbles, snacks – in the car at the desk
        by the bed by the telly. Junk food all day

STUDIOSE
Masterchef jus julienne foam fondue caramelise clarify
concentrate Nigella blanch barbecue Maggie Beer marinate
Gordon Ramsay grate grind smash smoke smother stuff souflé
puree pulverise whip to unwavering peaks *My Kitchen Rules*

St Alphonsus Liguori
It is a defect to eat like beasts, with the sole motive of sensual gratification

LAUTE
    saffron sugared flower petals rose oil edible gold gooseberry barnacles abalone panko breadcrumbs krill oil chia seeds wagyu beef caviar Caciocavallo Podolico *foie gras* truffles

St Gregory the Great
The irregular desire is the sin not the food

PRAEPROPERE
    Food on the run, brekkie in a drink,
    lunch at the desk, drive through,
    take away, food to go, graze all day.

St Alphonsus Ligori
The most delicious meats can be eaten without sin if the motive be good and worthy and of a rational creature. Taking the coarsest food through attachment to pleasure is committing a sin.

ARDENTE
    If we don't eat between meals, or eat too much
    the hungrier we are, and the more eager we'll be for
    the next meal. So if we obey all the other exhortations
    we'll necessarily disobey this one.

So who shall win the fight for our souls?
The Beast or the Priest?

Removing the Christ…

1

Ho Ho Ho food – heavy, hearty, hot –
Golden roast and steaming pud
brandy sauce, crispy pastry
sweet and spicy groggy soggy
crumbly buttery sugary shortbread
cinnamon, cloves, raisins, allspice

Orange and lemon and brandy and wine
brandy crumbly raisin steaming
orange and claret and ham and turkey
cranberries cinnamon allspice sugar
butter and butter and butter and cream
chook and duck and turkey and goose

Chestnuts and Yule log and boars head
(or ham) fruit cake and fruit mince
pastry and ice cream and brandy and cream
bread sauce cranberry sauce brandy sauce
shortbread (meltingly buttery creamery sugary)
candy canes sugar and sugar and jolly red food colouring

2

The wonder of winter
with the swirling of snow
the frosted-up windows with icicle art
clutches of carollers swath-ed in fur
twinkling of candles, pungent of pine

breath steaming, foot stamping
nose dripping, wool fingered
Come in by the fire!
Oh for a friendly fire, welcoming, beckoning…

Ours glowers in mountains
Our smoke's in the air
A strange orange sun blisters the sky
Forty degrees and it's nine in the morning
Water the garden before they wake up
Then the excited crackle of opening the pressies
the slurping of mangoes, the fizz of champagne

Are we really going to turn on the oven?

3

You can't cut out Christ
Let's talk about symbols:
Our rounded mince pies
were once large and square
the crib in the manger!
And the marzipan stollen
all white and rounded
like a bundle of baby…

And then there's plum pudding
with its thirteen ingredients:
they are the guests at that vital Last Supper
Stir that pudding from east to west
and you follow the path of those very wise men
bearing their gifts of exotic spices –
nutmeg, cinnamon, allspice, cloves
all in our cake – which should only
be eaten on 12th night
when they finally arrived in Bethlehem

4

More or less reason to follow tradition?
Can we really cut the strings of that apron?
And have festive food for atheist Aussies
prawns and pavs in a tent on the beach
Cold chook by the river, sipping a beer
while squealing kids swing over and splash

Still a few nods – plum pudding ice cream;
the ubiquitous ham; Pagan not Christian

(used to be boar's head, tribute to Freja!)
Mangoes and peaches, apricots, cherries
Why all that dried fruit when it's fresh off the tree?

So a toast to the holidays, families and friendship –
beaches and barbecues, bushfire free
a snip of that apron and one day soon –
Christ Almighty!
an Aussie Republic…

Comfort Food

1 Hot chips

When perfect they are the epitome
       of 'blisspoint'
              crispy outside meltyinside
                      salt and fat in perfect combination
They have to be hot!
Nothing worse than a cold soggy chip…

Best eaten in the car
       on a freezing day
              rain pounding down
                      windows fogged
Eaten straight from the paper
licking the salt from your fingers
                you're as warm inside, as it is cold out

2 Crumpets

With lots of butter and 'Cocky's Joy'*
       that musky sweetness oozing from the holes
              more sticky finger licking

Best eaten by the fire
       napkin at neck.
              paper towels at the ready
accompanied by a hot chocolate
or a rum toddy

3 Boiled eggs with 'soldiers'

My friend calls this 'nursery food'
       of course when you cut your toast
              into straight strips like ramrod soldiers…
But there is nothing better to eat with one of your
chicken's gifts –
              soft boiled with salt and black pepper
              even a dab of butter!
Best eaten with a nice cup of tea

4 Hot Cross buns (any time of the year)

The best thing about Easter
       is not white edged reconstituted chocolate
              little cocoa – largely sugar
It is the perfect hot cross bun
filled with fruit, spices and candied peel
              real flour, so they're not squashy

Not being Christian
I eat them all year
sometimes I make them
without the cross

Best eaten toasted with my own grapefruit marmalade
       (salute to Dad the marmalade maker!)
         the tangy citrus complimenting the spice and peel –
         and a good strong coffee

5 Borscht (like my Gran made)

She made it with red cabbage and beetroot
       still in big chunks (no pissy puree)
              sometimes some smoky rookwurst
always a swirl of sour cream – 'rose red with snow white'
as beautiful as it tastes

Best served on a cold winter night in white porcelain bowls
       with a hunk of rye bread
       and of course, a good red

6 Baguette with home-cured salami and chèvre

Discovered on my first trip to France
       when as a poor student
              it was most of my meals
And who could want for more?
The crunch of the bread, the creamy saltiness of the chèvre
and the salty garlicky umami salami…

Best eaten as an occasional guilty pleasure
       (now we know what's good for us)
       on a picnic rug in a park with a cheap red in a plastic cup –
       the taste of nostalgia

* Cocky's Joy – Australian slang for golden syrup

13 things I've learned from Diets – (and one extra)

Our diet has five components – protein, fat, carbohydrates, fruit and vegetables. There is a pyramid. Every few years the pyramid inverts

Protein and carbohydrate are digested in different parts of the stomach so shouldn't be eaten together

Fruit should only be eaten on its own and first thing in the morning, and if you are cutting out carbs, the only fruit allowed are berries, and only in season

Grapefruit and pineapple contain an enzyme that helps burn body fat. Pineapple has the extra advantage of making you sexier, as in *The Sexy Pineapple diet*

Egg yolks are bad for you – too much fat. Eat only whites. Eggs are bad for you – too much cholesterol. Eat only one a week

A hard-boiled egg for breakfast is difficult to digest, so have one daily, and it will speed up your metabolism and help you lose weight

Don't drink water with meals as it's bad for digestion. (Obviously the answer is to drink wine instead.) Red wine is good for your heart.

The more you sleep the more weight you lose, as the time you are asleep you could be eating, as in *The Sleeping Beauty diet*

Because they lived healthy lives (we know by their medical records) – follow the example of paleo humans – eating only meat, nuts and berries in season.

We weren't meant to eat meat – our digestive system can't tolerate it
The existence of canines means we evolved to eat meat

You need to eat small regular meals to keep your metabolic fires stoked (as in the low GI diet)
You need to fast regularly to allow cells to rebuild themselves, (as in *The 2/5 Fast diet*)

If you cut out carbs and eat mainly protein and vegetables your body goes into ketosis, your body burns the fat that is usually stored, you lose lots of weight as in KETO diet

My friend told me if you eat a lot of Wagon Wheels, they weigh your body down and you lose weight carrying it around

*

Eat food,
Not too much,
Mainly from plants.

The Peasants – Spuds and Cabbage

All these interlopers – asparagus, artichoke
short seasons, high cost, hipster fads
kale smoothies! I ask you…

Don't forget us – the stayers, the salt
of the earth… Feeding the masses through all the long winters
when your delicate favourites are not to be found –

Protecting their precious princess personas
with their dramatic appearance in spring
but we're always here – solid, sustaining

Dependable! But so low on your list
we don't even warrant a separate poem…
We claim our own stanzas at least:

> Me – much maligned cabbage
> unpleasant echoes of squalor and smells
> boarding school kitchens and rooming house corridors
>
> Same cruciferous family
> as your trendy friend kale
> and just as good for you:
>
> protection from radiation; prevention of cancer;
> reduction of heart disease, blood pressure;
> optimises blood flow to the brain –
>
> So I help you stay sharp…
> And don't you remember the instant relief
> of cupping your football hard

milk swollen breasts, in my perfect curved leaves –
Add mastitis prevention to the list, as well as
a talking point for all those baby-glazed gawpers

> But sadly you and your tuberous mates
> are just a bit stodgy, and solo – quite tasteless
> edible only with garlic and bacon
>
> And you – humble spud
> are way too humble
> without at least butter and salt
> (cheese and cream if you're French)
>
> As one of the night-shades
> with your poisonous green tinges
> you can be malign – a killer no less
>
> And when you're grown on your own
> you can summon disease, famine
> when those you sustained are steadily starved…

Just your 'efficient agricultural practices'
We prefer a field with a variety of friends
And you are blind to our subtlety

Needing to smother us with salt and fat
Have you ever had us from soil to pot?
No need for any of your additives then

Really, could a Desiree or Toolangi Delight
be humble? Or the feisty Red Rascal or
spunky Spunta or sumptuous Yukon Gold…

And have you forgotten the deep satisfaction
the salty, crispy, lip and finger-licking joy
of hot chips on a freezing day…

But we'll wait patiently in our cold
cellars, disparaged, ignored, waiting
for you to tire of your fussy fads

and come back to earth…

Voracious needs mass production
Mass sales, mass seduction
Ensures the good stuff's for the wealthy
A few organic farms can keep them healthy

Spoon Feeding

Older people deserve the very best food, enticing and delicious meals that uplift and bring joy – Maggie Beer

Is it a joyous return
to the anarchy of id?
with their blubber and bibs
Gaa gaa mother feed me…

More grey sludge, more, more…
That's enough
Jaws clamp shut
Grey dribble down chin

At the close of the circle
in a world where
to be young is to be
To be old is not

Patronised tolerated
At best
Worse still
Ignored, abused

They're on their way out
Don't know the difference
No point wasting…
Let them eat shit

*

Marvellous Maggie
Nearly eighty, testimony
To her Good Food crusade…

Recipes for Life 　　　　　*Blueberry, chia and*
Foods to combat dementia　　*coconut smoothie*
Cholesterol, diabetes

Jewel coloured, delicious　　*Smoked trout salad*
Balanced, nutritious　　　　*with grilled peaches*
Bury that grey sludge!　　　*and rocket*

Maggie Beer Foundation　　*Pan-fried whiting*
Training cooks and chefs　　*with celery and*
To make 'food for life'　　　*pomegranate*

In the dens of despair　　　*Spelt pappardelle*
Where grey sludge　　　　 *with pumpkin, sage*
Was king　　　　　　　　*and walnuts*

We lose sight, sound　　　 *Chicken and chickpea*
And taste　　　　　　　　*tagine with turmeric*
Such a need to entice

*

But it's part of the plan   *Coconut pannacotta*
We eat less as we move less   *with raspberries*
Shrink a bit   a*nd toasted almonds*

Like a toddler
Jaws clamp shut
Close the circle

In the end
It gives us power
No more

Voracious (2)

Seeds of Destruction

tiny seedlings / family farms / farmer's markets / Yes!
to recycling bins green bags / No! to battery chickens
plastic bags / fracking coal / *Lock the Gate!*

War on Waste /our 'David' / Rucastle / the hero!
supermarkets become magnanimous / forced / to give away
'waste' to the needy / freegans dumpster-divers / help themselves

mother earth herself / protests / earth fire water air
quakes bushfires hurricanes cyclones / tsunamis tornados floods
Gaia vs Voracious… / now they'll learn / *won't they?*

Gaia says not enough / let's try plague / slow down shut down start again
rethink essential / make / grow / borrow / steal / shopping
becomes scary / QR codes tier 1 hot spots / no fun / any more

do it less often / check the fridge / reign in greed / rethink need
Voracious groans / getting thin / suffering from / this nonconsumption
diet / can't survive / without accumulation / getting thinner / fading away…

you wish / no Moses and the profits / but still inequality
haves can afford change / organic and markets and handmade
and local / still too dear / for those at the bottom / products always

much cheaper / than produce / people in high rise / no room
to grow / people in factories /no time / to bake
junk food's the cheapest / and so addictive…

He's still here / if surly / swatting at all / those tiny brave Davids
though the first / was alone / Goliath a pushover / compared to our boy
he's so adaptive / *oh I can renew* / *I'll make green sexy*

after all / if it makes me more money…
We need a whole system / to wipe out Voracious
rejecting the notion/ of profit as king / our hope is the young ones

Extinction Rebellion! they voted for socialism / for Bernie and Jeremy
just to get close / gives cause to hope /people are thinking
and knowledge is power

and it all starts / with one / tiny seed…

www.ingramcontent.com/pod-product-compliance
Lightning Source LLC
Chambersburg PA
CBHW071023080526
44587CB00015B/2468